SECRETS OF CRYSTAL HEALING:

A Beginner's Guide to Healing the Natural W[orld]

Miriam Petersen

Table of Contents

Additionally, the information in the following pages is intended only for informational purposes and should thus be thought of as universal. As befitting its nature, it is presented without assurance regarding its prolonged validity or interim quality. Trademarks that are mentioned are done without written consent and can in no way be considered an endorsement from the trademark holder.

Introduction

Thank you for taking the time to download this book: Secrets of Crystal Healing: A Beginner's Guide to Healing the Natural Way.

For millennia, humans have been harnessing the power of crystals in ritual and healing. From the ancient Sumerians (who used quartz in their magic rituals) to the Greeks (who believed that the power of hematite would make them invulnerable in battle) and the Egyptians (who protected themselves from evil spirits and night terrors with peridot and topaz), the use of crystals in aiding humanity is well-documented. Indeed, the use of crystals for healing can be traced to the fabled island of Atlantis!

Crystals continue to serve humanity to this day. Look up and you will likely see an LCD screen near you. What you may not have realized is that "LCD" stands for "Liquid Crystal Display." Silicon, of Silicon Valley fame and one of the main components in your computer's motherboard, is derived from quartz crystal. Thus, crystals continue to be essential to humanity to this day.

My journey into the world of crystal healing started 5 years ago. At the time, I was deeply dissatisfied with my life and was seeking something more. I was suffering from anxiety and felt depressed. While I believe and support the use of clinical medicine in our modern society, I wanted to explore other forms of aid to address the intangible. I began investigating holistic and alternative medicines and, in these explorations, discovered a whole new world of healing waiting to be brought back into the light.

I am delighted to share with you the secrets of crystal healing. In the following pages, you will learn about what a crystal is, the history of crystal healing, how to choose crystals for your specific ailments, and how to cleanse and program crystals for your needs. My hope is, at the end of this book, you will have a good understanding of how to harness the power of crystals and utilize them for your health and happiness.

Once again, thanks for downloading this book. I hope you find it to be helpful!

Chapter 1
What Is Crystal Healing?

Crystal healing is an alternative form of medicine and healing that harnesses the power of crystals and other precious and semi-precious stones to cure and prevent illnesses. At the very core of this entire system of therapy is the idea that different crystals have different vibrations. By interfacing with your personal electromagnetic field, crystals can channel healing energy into your body. When used properly, crystals can serve as a conduit to the nurturing power of the earth, repairing and rebuilding your health and energy, while detoxifying your body of negativity, and shielding you against electromagnetic pollution. Crystals can also be used to purify your home and other spaces. Elements of crystal healing have been used in meditation, Reiki, spirit healing, and massage therapy.

To embrace crystal healing is to invite a beautiful method of self-healing and personal power into your life. It is not only a non-invasive and holistic, but cures both the body and the mind. Crystal healing helps give a physical remedy in a holistic way, and it is also beneficial when it comes to taking control of the mind. It boosts confidence and brings out the positive persona of the practitioner. It wards off negativity and infuses one with positive energy. Crystal healing can help people regain their lost balance, which is a common source of many kinds of misery.

In many ways, it relies on your sense of purpose and intentionality. While crystals are extremely powerful in their own right, you must use them with intent and purpose to fully utilize their healing vibrations. Essentially, crystals hold your intent and remind you of your connection to the Earth. Therefore, whether you are focusing the power of crystals through a crystal grid or programming a crystal pendant to wear against your skin, or simply putting a crystal beneath your pillow when you sleep, you must do so with a strong sense of purpose. Your intent is the foundation from which your crystals draw their strength. You must *believe* in the healing, nourishing power of crystals wholeheartedly and act with intention when harnessing that power-without a strong sense of belief, it loses all efficacy.

An Enduring Enigma

While it might seem baffling to people who are analyzing it from a distance, crystal healing is hailed for its curative powers by those who practice it. When you begin your journey into the world of crystal healing, it is easy to become overwhelmed by the names of the multitude of crystals, by the different methodologies, and by the sheer power and opportunity it offers. However, it is a rewarding path to walk and you will soon be able to converse upon the topic with authority.

As we touched upon in the introduction, the use of crystals in healing goes back to antiquity. Jet beads, bracelets, and necklaces were found in Belgiam gravesites dating back to the Paleolithic Era. Ancient amulets made of amber were found in Britain, dating back 30,000 years. The use of crystals in magic rites were found inscribed on ancient Sumerian tablets. Egyptian pharaohs used semi-precious stones, including lapis lazuli, carnelian, turquoise, clear quartz, and emerald, to focus their judgement and to ward off evil.

It was the ancient Greeks who truly codified the different uses for different crystals. The word "crystal" is derived from the Greek word "πάγος" (pronounced 'págos'). The Greeks believed that clear quartz was water that had frozen so deeply that it would always remain solid. Hematite received its name from the Greek "αἱματίτης λίθος," or "blood-red stone," and was believed to have rendered one's flesh invulnerable in battle.

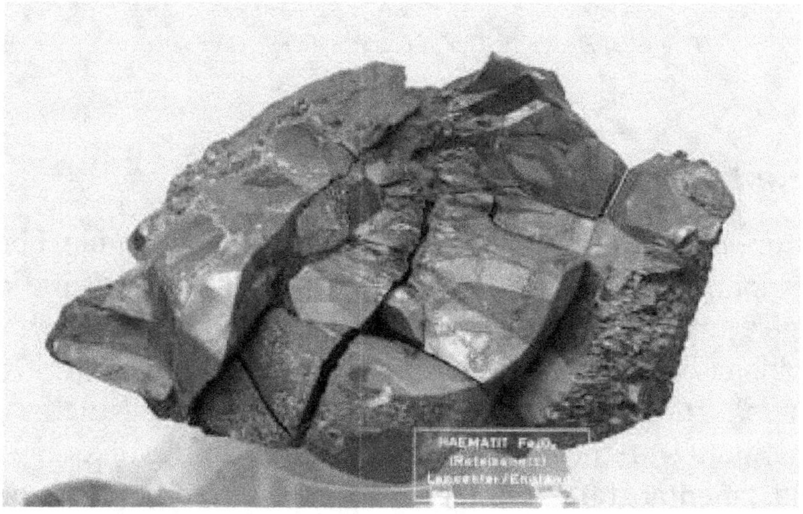

Figure 1: Hematite comes in a variety of colors, including black, silver gray, brown, or red.

Jade continues to hold great significance to this very day in China. Ancient Chinese emperors would bedeck themselves in jade, for its potent protective qualities and health benefits. In modern day China, it is believed that wearing a jade bracelet is to be protected from harm or injury. There are many anecdotes of how people who have survived grievous accidents have attributed their survival to the jade jewelry they wore at that time of the incident.

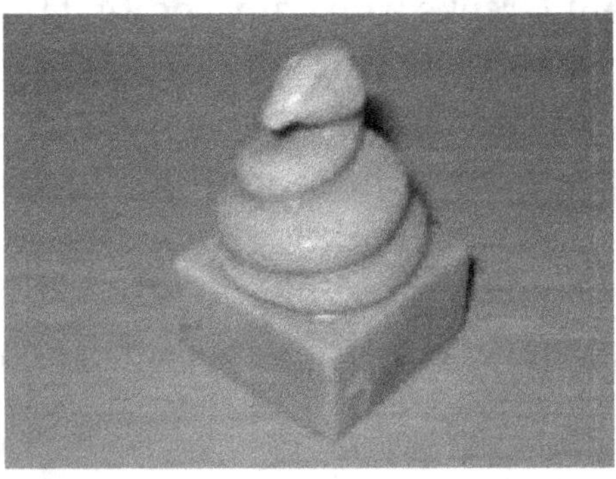

Figure 2: Jade is prized for its protective qualities and beauty.

Crystal Healing

Nature has done a wonderful job in creating the human body. It is complex yet coordinated. Every organ has its specific job, largely unrelated to the functions of the other organs. Yet problems in one organ will often affect the function of the others. There are tangible processes that regulate the functioning of the body. But intangible things like energy fields, mental state, and the environment also have an equal impact. Mankind is equally troubled by the problems of the mind as it is troubled by the problems of the body. Pain and suffering brought about by the imbalance of energy can be immense. Here, the keyword is "imbalance."

Crystal healing is the process of bringing balance to the person's energy. Science has proven that the world runs on energy. It has also proven that energy can neither be created nor destroyed. Imbalance of energy is the cause of all the commotion that takes place in this world. We could be talking about a steaming kettle or two large countries, it will be the same in both cases: whenever there is any disturbance, the main reason is the imbalance in energy or power. Crystals work as the pipeline through which energy balance can be established within your body, mind, and soul. It eases our pain and sufferings. We can let the buildup of negative energy flow out and the positive energy come. This will bring great relief.

How Does Crystal Healing Work?

Nature has blessed mankind with several gifts. Flora and fauna help us as our sustenance. The environment helps us in survival. The rivers, seas, and oceans provide water. The soil carries the minerals and energy that help in operating this world.

We, the mortal beings, are also parts of this Mother Earth. We are made up of simple constituents found on earth, and at the end of our lifespan, only the simpler things remain. Incidentally, crystals are also made up of those constituents. They have an added advantage. Earth took thousands of years to create crystals. They have endured a lot of pressure and heat. Some of them may have rested in their birthing place for hundreds of centuries. This makes them a storehouse of radiant energy—the same energy which can bring balance and cure illnesses.

Crystal healing is the science of understanding the problem areas in the body and the reasons behind those problems, as well as of finding the solutions. It strives to restore the energy balance in your body. It helps you in releasing the negative energy by activating your chakras and channeling the positive energy of the crystals into your body.

Crystals are amazing. They are completely natural and have passed the test of time, pressure, and heat. They have a perfect geometric formation. The color, size, mineral, and type of crystals can be different, but all possess one or the other type of energy. This energy can be used to heal you. The amount of energy a crystal holds will depend on its color, type, and placement. Crystal healing deals with understanding the problems and finding the right crystal for restoring the energy balance. It is the science of bringing harmony. The natural structure of the crystals can stabilize your emotions, psyche, and physical body systems. They stimulate us when it's needed, creating positive vibrations to bring order in the problem areas and aiding our efforts to heal our body without foreign aid.

Our body has a very efficient self-healing mechanism. The processes of degeneration and regeneration are continuous in our body. Cells take form, grow old, and die on a regular basis. We get injured, and the body immediately seeks to heal itself. But there are times when the injury or attack is more than our healing capacity could manage. There may come blows that are harder than we can bear—the pain more excruciating than we can endure. In such cases, the self-healing mechanism becomes sluggish, inefficient, or ineffective. The positive energy required to recover is deficient. Healing crystals can provide the required impetus in such cases. They have the power to influence the balance of energy in your body. Some crystals emit energy-lifting vibrations while others have a calming or soothing effect. The art is to identify the right crystals for the job and to know their placement.

The Placement

Each unique individual and situations would require different combinations of crystals. All crystals produce different kinds of effects. The amount of energy they would radiate will also depend on the crystal's size and on its color. Along with these, the placement of crystals and their use are also equally important. You may need crystals for bringing calm to your workplace. In that case, they need to be placed at strategic locations where they can work as a grid. If you are using crystals for relaxation, then their placement will be different.

You will have to understand the human energy field and its relationship with various chakras in our body. This will help you get the most out of crystals. A proper understanding of the human energy field comes from the understanding of the body chakras. They dictate the functioning of your body, and crystals can directly affect these chakras. If you know the art of activating the chakras and the crystals, then reaching harmony will become very simple.

The Chakras

From the top of the head where the Crown Chakra is placed to the base of your spine where the Root Chakra is placed, there are seven chakras. All chakras have their specific purposes and control important functions. Negative energy, toxins, pollution, and the corruption of the modern world are some of the problems that may lead to the blockage of these chakras. If blocked, these chakras can become unreceptive of energy and may cause physiological, mental, and spiritual disorders. You may feel a lack of spirit or interest. You may start falling sick often. Your immunity might go down. These are just some of the problems. Unblocking the chakras and refreshing them with the energy of these crystals can give you a new lease on life. It can rekindle your body, mind, and spirit. It will make you feel rejuvenated and re-energized.

The following chapters will give you insight into the chakras and their importance in healing. They'll also explain the various crystals that can be used for healing some of the common problems. You will also get to know about the importance of the placement of crystals when it comes to in healing. This book will tell you the ways to energize your crystals, along with all you need to know about crystal maintenance.

Chapter 2:
The Importance and Impact of Chakras

We all radiate energy. Some call it the "vibe;" others call it "aura" or "charisma." You may call it by any name, but it's all the same. It is something you can feel in one form or another when you encounter someone else. This energy comes from the chakras in our body. It affects us strongly. You will start feeling negativity when you are in the company of a person filled with negativity and pessimism. You will feel elated in the company of a kind and optimistic person despite your own mood. The company of leaders motivates you, and the company of followers makes you meek and submissive.

Everyone has seven chakras, or centers of energy. It is through those chakras that energy flows in and out of your body. These chakras also have a very strong impact on your ability to function and interact with others. They regulate your mood, actions, and thoughts. They can elevate your natural strengths but can also snatch it from you if you are out of balance. It is important to know these chakras.

The literal meaning of the word "chakra" is "wheel." These are the wheels of energy that drive our body, mind, soul, thoughts, feelings, and actions. They are very important as we are the sum of our thoughts and actions. An imbalance of energy in any chakra will lead to problems. Modern medical science tries to treat the symptoms. It has no way of treating the very problem itself because that is generally intangible. Crystal healing, in contrast, deals with the imbalance of energy in the chakras and targets the root of the problem, seeking to provide an effective solution.

To begin on your crystal healing journey, it is important to know first about the chakras and the problems that can arise when they are in a state of imbalance.

The Seven Chakras					
Name	Corresponding Color	Power	Problems Caused by Imbalance	Type of Stone	Color of Stone
The Root Chakra	Red	Brings stability, satiety, and focus	Fear and anxiety; constipation, obesity, osteoarthritis, and sexual problems	Calcite, Jasper, Garnet	Red and Black
The Sacral Chakra	Orange	Creativity, passion, emotions, and sexuality	Impotence, poor libido, constipation, muscle cramps; kidney, bladder, and urinary problems	Amber, Fossilized Tree Resin, Carnelian	Orange
The Solar Plexus Chakra	Yellow	Self-identity, humor, warmth, and confidence	Digestive issues; problems of the stomach, liver, pancreas, gallbladder, and diaphragm	Citrine, The Tiger's Eye, Topaz	Yellow
The Heart Chakra	Green	Love, affection, and forgiveness	Heart and lung problems; hypertension, asthma, and emotional issues	Emerald, Jade, Nephrite, Quartz	Green
The Throat Chakra	Turquoise	Communication and self-expression	Cold, stiff neck; hearing and voice problems; hyperthyroidism and back pain	Turquoise, Aquamarine	Blue
The Third Eye Chakra	Indigo	Psychic abilities, intuition,	Blurred vision, headache, hallucination	Amethyst, Quartz, Lapis Lazuli	Indigo

		knowledge, and concentration	, nightmares, and mental problems		
The Crown Chakra	Violet	Cosmic energy, thoughts, and imagination	Migraine, depression, and headache	Opalite, Ruby	White and Purple

As you can see from the table, these seven chakras dominate your functions and powers. Any blockage in these chakras can have a negative impact on your body and performance. You may start becoming indecisive, weak, and frail. These chakras control the physiological as well as the psychological aspects of your personality.

The Root Chakra

This is the base chakra. It is situated at the root of your spine. It keeps you grounded and satisfied. If there is a blockage in this chakra, then you will begin to experience problems regarding safety and security. Fear and anxiety will grip you and make you indecisive. You will feel unsatisfied, and you might question your identity. This chakra can be impacted by sudden traumatic changes in life like the death of a loved one or abandonment. You may face physiological problems like pain in the legs, feet, hips, knees, and ankles. Eating disorders, constipation, and diarrhea may also start troubling you. Water retention and lower back pain may also start to trouble you. Sexual problems may become a concern.

Feelings of depression and of being undeserving are the first ones to grip a person suffering from an imbalance in this chakra. Negative feelings like insecurity, indecisiveness, and phobia take precedence in the decision-making process. Negative energies get no release, and slowly, paranoia starts taking control.

Crystals and chakra stones like Garnet, Red Zincite, Red Jasper, Smokey Quartz, Black Tourmaline, and Black Obsidian are helpful for bringing back balance.

The Sacral Chakra

This chakra dominates sensuality, creativity, and emotions. Located in the lower abdomen, this is the chakra that controls your pleasures and indulgences. It brings fluidity of thoughts and emotions. Problems in this chakra can lead to restrictions in the expression of sexuality and sensuality. Physical symptoms including a lowered libido and lack of pleasure in sexual activity are very prominent. Eating disorders and obesity are also very common problems caused by the imbalance in this chakra. Problems in conception, irregular menstrual cycle, and miscarriages are also some of the serious consequences.

Psychological problems may include mood swings, creative blocks, and lack of joy. Sexual obsessions and indifference towards others may also arise. The Sacral Chakra can get blocked in people who were traumatized, neglected, or abused in their childhood. People with a blocked Sacral Chakra will suffer from self-esteem and anxiety issues. This leads to continuous efforts to please others, but the results are never satisfactory. Their relationships are short and unfulfilling.

Orange and blue-green stones and crystals like Carnelian, Orange Calcite, Turquoise, Fluorite, and Vanadite are very helpful when it comes to healing this chakra.

The Solar Plexus Chakra

This is the energy center of our body. This chakra is connected to our digestive system, so it makes sense that it is located in the upper abdomen. Your willpower, energy, and strength to achieve your goals are connected with it. (Think of the old saying, "No guts, no glory!") It makes you assertive and fierce.

The physiological problems arising due to problems in this chakra are the inability to concentrate or memorize important things. Intestinal and digestive problems are also common. Diabetes, obesity, skin diseases, ulcer, and chronic fatigue may also haunt the people suffering from an imbalance in this chakra. The psychological impact is also equally serious, if not more.

People with lower energy in this chakra may feel a lack of self-respect, phobia of attention, and lower self-esteem. They remain confused and indecisive, leading to poor life choices and a general lack of success. They easily lose control over situations and feel paralyzed.

However, high energy in this chakra is also equally problematic. It will lead to an inflated ego, extreme extroversion, and an abusive nature. They would also tend to get very manipulative and aggressive, causing problems for themselves and others.

Yellow-hued stones and crystals like Yellow Jasper, Golden Calcite, and Citrine are helpful in bringing back balance to this chakra.

The Heart Chakra

This is the chakra of love, compassion, and forgiveness. It is located in the center of your chest, as you would expect it to be. It establishes a connection between the physical and the spiritual world. Feelings of peace, joy, faith, hope, and belongingness are associated with this chakra. The physiological problems associated with problems in this chakra are pneumonia and asthma. People affected with it may also feel pain in the upper back and shoulders. Vertigo, heart diseases, and chest and breast problems are also common.

The psychological impacts of imbalance in this chakra are heartlessness and indifference. Unhappiness and lack of peace keep such people in the grip. They become over-possessive and face problems in trusting others. They are simply unable to count their blessings and would keep on blaming others. They become cold, indifferent, difficult, and aloof. Imbalance in this chakra will make a person very sad and bitter. They completely lose the capacity to receive love. Feelings of paranoia, confusion, and unworthiness grip them completely.

Pink and green stones and crystals like Tourmaline, Malachite, Aventurine, Rose Quartz, and Jade are very helpful for bringing balance to this powerful chakra.

The Throat Chakra

This is the chakra of communication and expression. Virtually based on the throat, this chakra gives voice to your thoughts. The main physiological symptoms denoting problems in this chakra are stuttering, hyperthyroidism, tonsillitis, and neck and shoulder pain. An imbalance may also make the victims lie frequently and needlessly. They choke on words and frequently feel a lump in their throat while talking. Voice problems and tone deafness are also some physiological problems associated with this chakra.

Psychologically, a blockage would greatly suppress the personality of the victim and will lead to social anxiety. One tends to develop a phobia of speaking in public and may have a hesitance with words. Extreme shyness and an inability to listen to others is also a clear symptom of the problem. Victims are not able to express themselves properly and also often break their promises. Frustration and restlessness are clear results of such problems. The victims become very timid, shy, and face problems in coping with society.

Blue and light blue stones and crystals like Angelite, Kyanite, Turquoise, Sodalite, and Calcite are very helpful for restoring balance to this chakra.

The Third Eye Chakra

This is the chakra of awareness and foresight. Located between and slightly above the eyes, it brings the powers of imagination, intuitiveness, and psychic intuition together. It gives you the power of insight and wisdom. You can establish a deep connection with yourself and with the world if this chakra is balanced. However, an energy imbalance in this chakra will lead to physiological symptoms like eye disorders, insomnia, headaches, hallucinations, and hair loss. The psychological impact is even deeper, and the victim may become confused in most situations and lose clarity. Illogical fear and close-mindedness are also very common. Victims lose their sense of time and tend to become very pessimistic in nature.

This is a very powerful chakra as it controls the vision of the world and the ability to sense and perceive threats. The victim will become very difficult and insecure. Decisions will start going wrong due to the short-sightedness. It will seem as if the whole world is conspiring against the victim. They feel a sense of victimization and developing a non-assertive personality that's unsure of their own abilities is a common trait among these individuals.

Purple, dark blue, and indigo stones and crystals like Azurite and Lapis Lazuli are very helpful in restoring balance to this chakra.

The Crown Chakra

This is the chakra of consciousness and cosmic energy. Sensibly located on your crown, or the top of your head, it connects you with the universe and unifies you with the greater powers of the cosmos. It gives you clarity of mind, wisdom, and consciousness. The main physiological problems associated with the imbalance in this chakra are nervous system and neurological problems. The victim may develop an unusual sensitivity to light and may have constant headaches. Auto-immune disorders and mental disorders such as schizophrenia are also associated with this imbalance. The evident psychological problems associated with it are the sense of utter confusion, helplessness, and disorientation. People suffering from it also lose faith and develop a lot of fears. They become apathetic or indifferent. Fear and depression grip them. Depression, migraines, and headaches may become common affairs for the victims.

Golden-white and violet crystals like Amethyst, White Calcite, and White Topaz are very helpful in restoring the balance of energy to this chakra.

Chapter 3: Healing by Crystals

Crystal healing can be used for easing the pain of mind, body, and soul. It leads the energies in your body to synchronize. It restores harmony and makes you at peace. A person with an agitated body and mind is always restless, unable to enjoy the ultimate pleasures. They can be likened to tourist guides who boast of the marvels of a place to tourists but find no pleasure in them at all. All the toil in the world becomes worthless when you lose the taste to enjoy them. It becomes a sordid tale.

Crystal healing is very helpful in regaining the balance of energy so that you can enjoy the pleasures you sought so hard for. It makes you full of vigor and vitality as your power to both consume and give returns.

Physical Healing

Physical pain and suffering are usually the most apparent. You can feel it as acutely as the people around you can see it. Mainstream medical science has made tremendous progress in healing physical pain and suffering. There are innumerable medicines, antibiotics, painkillers, treatments, and surgeries to ease the pain and suffering borne by us. However, there are side effects too. There are such things as drug abuse, overuse, and insensitivity. The problems emerge, subside, and relapse. Many problems go away temporarily but resurface quickly. There are immunity issues and problems related to vigor and vitality. These may appear to be the effect of problems in some of the other organs, but they may actually be indicating that the body is out of balance. Your body is pleading for balance to be restored and is sending you signals to this end.

Crystal healing can help you regain this balance without having to be exposed to medicines and surgeries, but crystal healing doesn't ask you to stop your medication or treatment. It is an alternative treatment process that strives to heal you internally. It tries to restore the energy balance. It has no side effect and gives great relief.

Examples of Physical Ailments Crystal Healing Can Help

Arthritis

Arthritis in itself is very painful. It usually comes at a time when age is not on your side, and that can multiply the pain. To add further salt to injury, there is no specific cure for it medically. The pain steadily increases with time and keeps making daily life difficult with the passing seasons.

Crystal healing can be of great help in easing arthritic pain. It can give you relief while also healing you internally. Millions of people are suffering from arthritis globally, writhing in pain from this painful degeneration without respite, and healing crystals can be of great use to them.

You can use healing crystals in a number of ways to ease the arthritic pain. Meditating with healing crystals will help you to come out of the shadows of the crippling pain. You can wear the crystals for overall relief. Placing the crystals on your root chakras or the affected joints will give great ease.

Some of the crystals that can help you in this condition are:

Malachite

This beautiful green-colored healing crystal is a great strengthener. It helps in reducing inflammation and swelling in your body, which are the main causes of arthritic pain. However, care must be taken to keep the crystal in a sealed state. Broken malachite can release dust that can cause palpitation of the heart.

Blue Lace Agate

This soothing and beautiful light-blue stone has a calming effect. It is very helpful for arthritic pain as it eases the pain and gives great relief. This stone, which comes in several shades of blue and purple, has a very soothing impact. Apart from arthritic pain, people with anger management issues would also benefit from bearing this stone. You can hold this stone in your hand while meditating to get extra relief from pain. The soothing energy from the stone will help in relaxing your over-inflamed joints.

Migraines

For all practical purposes, a migraine is simply a headache, albeit more extreme. But considering it as just another inconvenience is not an option for the victim. It can bring down even giants for days. It is one of the most difficult problems to treat as it lies in the most complicated part of the body, the brain. Besides debilitating pain, the victim may also face nausea, vomiting, speaking difficulties, numbness, and sensitivity to light and sound. A migraine can occur due to the imbalance in power or the blockage of the Third Eye Chakra and the Crown Chakra. Without treatment, the migraine will worsen from moderate to severe with the passing time. Sadly, allopathic medicine offers no permanent cure for migraines. It falls under the category of things that modern science is still discovering. However, alternative procedures like meditation and crystal healing offer great help. Along with your medication for migraine, practicing crystal healing can ease the intensity of the pain.

Some of the crystals that help in easing migraine are:

Amethyst

This is one of the most powerful healing stones. This beautiful purple quartz crystal brings balance to the violet flame of the Third Eye. It brings harmony to the sixth chakra and helps in easing the migraine. It also has other strong qualities like easing off addictions and shedding vices. This powerful stone infuses spiritual energy in your home. Keeping it under the pillow helps give one a sound sleep while keeping it in your home, in general, will bring protection. It is widely available and very purposeful, and it has the properties to establish energy balance in many other chakras as well.

Jet

This black energy-retaining stone has immense healing and protective abilities. It also has superb calming abilities that can help one deal with migraine pain, as well as pain from other parts of your body. The older the jet becomes, the more powerful it grows.

Lapis Lazuli

This is the blue stone of the psychics—beautiful to behold, bearer of great powers. It can mend the imbalance of power in the Third Eye Chakra that's causing the migraine. Not only that, but it can also help in improving the functioning of that chakra. If you are trying to open your third eye chakra, this is the stone for you.

Rose Quartz

This is the crystal of calmness, compassion, and creativity. It will help you ease the migraine pain. It works wonders with the Lapis Lazuli crystal as it accentuates the power of the other.

Migraines are generally caused by the energy blocks in the chakras. This makes regular cleansing of the crystals imperative. With time, the crystals tend to accumulate negative energy while they heal. Cleansing the crystals will help remove the negative energy, recharging it again in the process.

Skin Problems

Our skin is the cloth our body wears. It protects us from several kinds of infections and diseases, and we as a species attach great importance to its beauty. Its tone, softness, and color are a major cause of concern for the better half of the world's population. But it bears the brunt of extreme weather conditions, smoldering heat, and chilling winters. Allergies and infections also attack the skin easily due to high exposure. Even in ages past, when mankind knew little of medical science and skincare was the least of our concern, we still paid attention to it, and some civilizations have been putting healing crystals to that use from that time on. Healing crystals for skin issues serve a dual purpose. First, they protect the epidermis from the effects of the weather, and second, they can be used as ornaments to adorn its wearer.

The following are examples of skin problems and the healing crystals that could help with them:

Moonstone (Dry Skin)

Dry skin is one of the most common issues that concern people, especially those who live in places with cold, unfavorable climates. The skin loses the ability to hydrate itself and starts developing dry patches and filthy-looking cracks. With age, the skin starts losing elasticity and hydration. Healing crystals can help in restoring the elasticity and rehydration process, and moonstone is among the most powerful stones for this job. It replenishes the energy levels, rejuvenates, and rehydrates the skin.

Agate (Eczema)

This skin problem can make life difficult. Constant scratching, blisters, red patches, and rough scales are some of the problems caused by eczema. There are times when even the use of harsh steroids yields no result. Agate is a stone popularly used for healing and protection. It is beneficial for the heart and for blood circulation. It also heals emotional disharmony and improves the operations of the mind. You can wear it as a pendant and keep the crystal near your heart for best results. It will give great relief from itchy and flaky eczema.

Mental Healing

The human mind has been and is still an enigma for scientists and for humanity in general. So much has been discovered about its workings, yet there is so little that we know about its functioning. We are still not utilizing the full potential of our mind even though we have now been using it for millennia in this relatively developed state. It is the most difficult part of the body to perform surgeries on. As a hub of information, it has the power to coordinate, command, stimulate, and emulate. This one body part makes us superior to other beings on the planet. All that we have achieved and will achieve will surely be credited to this vital organ. Yet think of the unfortunate ones who are unable to use their mind even in its normal capacity. Think of the tragedy that they may be facing when it comes to treading their paths in the world.

There are several mental problems for which medical science is yet to find a definite answer. ADHD, Alzheimer's and Parkinson's disease, bipolar disorder, and insomnia are just some of the ailments that have no definite cures, or none that is very effective. Crystal healing can supplement your ongoing treatment, allowing you to get extra relief.

Some of the mental conditions crystal healing can help, and the relevant crystals for these conditions, are as follows:

ADHD

Attention deficit hyperactivity disorder (ADHD) leads to impulsive behavior and focus issues. There is no sure-fire cure for the disease, and the doctors can provide symptomatic treatment at best. What makes things worse is that 3-5% of children born in the USA suffer from this mental disorder, and most have to struggle throughout their lives due to this.

Crystal healing can come to your rescue if your child is also suffering from this problem. ADHD occurs due to the imbalance of energy in the sixth chakra, the Third Eye. This chakra is directly associated with the pineal gland and the hypothalamus. You can use several healing crystals to encourage improvement in your child's behavior.

Some of the important healing crystals to this end are:

Lepidolite

This purple crystal with white and black specks is among the most important crystals in healing problems of the mind. It works best on the Third Eye Chakra. This powerful crystal has such a strong calming effect that you can feel its power by simply holding it in your hand. It is used to heal a number of mental disorders like depression, stress, anxiety, insomnia, and bipolar disorder, along with ADHD. It is full of positive vibrations and helps in bringing life back in tune.

In people suffering from ADHD, this crystal stimulates the brain and improves its ability to think rationally. This prevents impulsive actions. It relaxes the mind and helps in decreasing the hyperactive nature of the patient.

Charoite

This is the stone that increases awareness and reduces fear and anxiety. This beautiful polished stone comes with hints of purple, white, and black. It boosts confidence and belief in oneself. It erases limiting beliefs and improves the thought process.

Fluorite

This pretty yellow crystal plays a crucial role in improving concentration abilities in people suffering from ADHD. It also boosts productivity and creativity. It works best on the Third Eye Chakra. You can use it with the other crystals for best effect.

Sodalite

This beautiful white stone has the power to stimulate thoughts and control feelings. It works wonders for people prone to panicking.

Lapis Lazuli

This stone is good for increasing concentration with the other gifts it brings. It improves creativity and communication as well. The darker blue shades of the crystal are better in helping with ADHD.

Bipolar Disorder

This is a rare brain disorder that has no medical cure. It is currently the most diagnosed mental disorder that affects more than 2.8% of the adult population in the US directly, with the people associated with them being affected indirectly. Its victims suffer from extreme and sudden mood shifts. The journey from ultra joyful to utterly hopeless may take only a few minutes, and before people can recover from the shock, the victim may have another mood shift again. Managing work and life become next to impossible for such people due to these sudden mood swings. They may remain depressed and sad for long stretches of time, and this makes maintaining steady relationships difficult as bouts of depression can last for weeks or even months. Such people may also have bouts of impulsiveness and euphoria, making them difficult for others to understand. They might have difficulty in sleeping and may also develop suicidal tendencies.

As said earlier, there is no definite cure for bipolar disorder. It can make the life of the person suffering from it very difficult. Alienation from society, depression, suicidal thoughts, and recurring failures become their fate. Crystal healing offers great help for this disease. Third Eye Chakra dominates the area of the brain causing this disorder. You can get relief by bringing back energy balance to this chakra. Specific crystals can help you in relieving the symptoms, which can resolve the problem to a great extent.

Some of the healing crystals for treating bipolar disorder are:

Lepidolite

This purple crystal works great with the Third Eye Chakra. It helps in reducing depression and emotional stress. It also helps in dealing with insomnia, addiction, stress, anxiety, and fear, as well as in controlling the fight-or-flight response to situations.

Kunzite

This pink crystal brings peace to life. It controls your anger and improves your interaction with people.

Charoite

This stone helps you fight fear and anxiety. It removes the limiting thoughts from your mind and widens your perspective. It will also make the bearer feel more energetic while also preventing energy pilferage.

Peridot

This crystal reduces unnecessary stress on the mind and brings harmony in life. It also helps fight feelings of jealousy and anger. It prevents the buildup of negative energies in the body. This green crystal boosts confidence and patience. It also works great on the Solar Plexus Chakra.

Spiritual Healing

Spiritual health is equally important for peace in life. Stress, anxiety, and problems with oneself and with others keep troubling us. They burden our conscience and spirit. Our karma also comes to haunt us and steals our peace. All these things blemish our spirit.

We carry a lot of baggage of the past on our backs. This blocks us from connecting with the higher consciousness. At one point or another, every individual feels the need to interact with the greater self, but such blockages can get in the way. Crystal healing can help you in attaining your spirituality. It enhances your psychic gifts and protects you against psychic attacks. Some crystals also help you heal wounds from the past life.

We carry a slate that needs to be wiped clean to balance the wheel of karma. It is a tough task, but imperative. You will need all the help you can get to do this. Crystal healing is one of them. It sharpens your intuition and clairvoyance. It protects you from the impact of negative energies around you, and it helps in your spiritual development.

Some of the stones that help in spiritual healing are:

Agate

This crystal can help you meditate. It enhances your meditation time and increases your focus. This crystal is also very helpful in linking you with the collective consciousness. It brings your thoughts and spirit into harmony, allowing you to start rediscovering peace within.

Amethyst

This crystal is helpful in many situations, but its contribution to spiritual healing is immense. This is the protector. It prevents you from psychic attacks and negative energies. It also enhances your psychic gifts and power of intuition.

Ametrine

When you seek the connection of your spirit with the higher consciousness, this crystal plays a very crucial role. It brings the physical and spiritual in sync.

Anhydrite

The wounds of the past have a karmic impact on your present. They prevent your spiritual awakening. This crystal helps in healing the past wounds.

Aquamarine

This crystal gives you the gift of sharp intuition and vision. It protects you from negative energies.

Azeztulite

This crystal helps in spiritual awakening. It raises your vibrational frequencies and helps in opening your Third Eye Chakra as well as the Crown Chakra.

Boji Stone

This stone brings harmony to your seven chakras. It aligns them and prepares the way for consciousness. When all the chakras start working in sync, attaining peace becomes very easy. It grounds you well and seals the energy leaks in your energy field.

Calcite

This crystal cleans your energy field and amplifies it. It balances the chakras and improves your psychic abilities.

Celestite

This is a high-vibration crystal that helps in meditation and in the opening of the Third Eye Chakra.

Charoite

This crystal promotes spiritual insight and also helps in opening and balancing the crown chakra.

Iolite

It helps in energizing the aura and in opening the third eye.

Jade

It is a protector crystal. It also helps in finding your spiritual path.

Kunzite

It is a high-vibration crystal that can stimulate you. It helps in meditation and also protects you from the influence of negative energies. This crystal aids in healing and understanding past life experiences. It brings your Heart Chakra in line with the Third Eye Chakra and Crown Chakra.

Malachite

This crystal amplifies your energy and clears and activates your chakras.

There are many more crystals that play some role or another in spiritual healing. The work of crystals is to aid your efforts. The important thing is to keep the efforts sincere and to use the stones wisely. They provide energy and bring balance to your chakras, but to achieve spiritual healing in the truest sense, the effort would have to be made by you.

Chapter 4:
How to Begin Using Crystals

You have learned about the healing power of crystals and their connection with the chakras. Now, it is time to address the question of how to use them to get the desired benefits. Crystals hold great power, and they can be used to heal. They will soothe and provide relief. Before that, however, the crystals will need to be prepared, cleaned, programmed, and activated. This chapter will share with you the ways of doing so.

There are many paths one can take to reach the same place. The way doesn't matter as much as the intent does. You will need to have belief. You will need to place your trust in the powers of the crystals to provide relief. Belief has great powers. It gives strength and fills you with energy. It opens your heart and makes you receptive. For crystal healing, you will need to become receptive.

The world is full of critics, some of whom are people who insist on having an opinion on anything and everything whether they have knowledge on the subject or not. Listening to every opinion will not help. Healing is a matter of great trust. When you believe in something, its power increases.

In Hinduism, there is a practice called "Pran Pratishtha." This is when people install stone statues in temples and, after performing rituals, start praying to them as if they're deities. To these people, the idol ceases to be a mere stone statue. They start believing that it is a representation of God. This practice is not exclusive to the Hindus. Be it a sacred book, statue, or another religious artifact of any religion in the world, as soon as people put their faith in it, the object rises above its original form and attains energy. It is not the object itself that has power but the faith placed in it.

Modern science questions crystal healing based on proof. Pitted against hard logic, any argument can become baseless. Healing and trust don't work that way. O. Henry's masterpiece story "The Last Leaf" is very apt for people who call crystal healing a bluff.

In the story, a girl survived the fight between life and death that had been anchored upon the falling of the last leaf of a maple tree. Her health had no connection with the falling of the leaves. Yet she believed that the tree was shedding the leaves at the same rate that her health was failing. She believed that she would also pass away on the day the last leaf of the tree falls. Slowly, all the leaves from the tree fell, except one. Strong winds blew, but that last leaf survived every challenge. She had almost given up on the hope of life, but she gained strength watching that last leaf braving the winds. She had established a connection with it. It gave her hope, and she started making attempts to regain her lost health. She rekindled the fighting spirit she had lost, and she recovered.

Hope can do wonders. Faith in powers unknown does give strength. It rekindles your spirit's will to fight and heals you. It is the same case with most alternative healing practices. Crystal healing has been in existence for thousands of years. It has been healing people when other treatment methods didn't yet exist. It isn't witchcraft. It is a practice that helps in healing. The world cannot doubt the simple fact that all matter is made up of energy—everything radiates some form of it. Our building blocks and the building blocks of crystals are the same; therefore, the transfer of energy stored in these crystals is not only possible but also helpful. We even use these minerals in various medicines. Crystal healing is a process that is based on receiving the healing powers through energy transfer in place of direct ingestion.

1. Choosing the Crystal

The first step toward crystal healing is finding the right crystals for yourself. Every aspect in this step is important and has meaning. Look up the problem that troubles you. Find its connection to the energy chakras in your body, and seek the type of stone that will help in healing that problem. Find the color of the stone that best fits the role you need to perform. Every part of this step is important.

If you are already suffering from some problem and there has been a diagnosis, then you already know what kind of healing to look for. If you don't know the real problem and you are seeking energy point activation, then you can begin by first activating your root chakra before moving up the scale. You must know the chakra you need to put your focus on. This will make your journey easier.

2. Cleansing the Crystals

Cleansing the crystals is an important task. This is a task which will have to be done on a regular basis. You must understand that crystals retain energy. There will be a regular exchange of energies, positive as well as negative. Therefore, it is a requirement to cleanse them before and after every use to keep them free from blockage. In this way, you will be able to get the most out of their potential. If you've bought them or have been gifted some crystals, then a thorough cleansing will be needed first and foremost to get rid of negative energies. You will need to purify them before putting them to use. The cleansing procedures are fairly simple and do not require special efforts.

Water Cleansing

Like other natural things, you can easily clean the crystals with water. Simply place your crystals under running tap water for 10 to 20 minutes. This will free them of impurities and negative energy. Although the best way is to put them underwater in a running stream like a river or a lake as it is the most natural method, it might not be convenient for everyone. If that's the case for you, the running water from the faucet of your own sink suffices.

Care should be taken that the water isn't hot. Heat can damage some crystals. The same goes for saltwater, or water laden with chemicals. Both can interfere with the chemical composition of the crystals and must, therefore, be avoided.

Sunlight and Moonlight Cleansing

In this cleansing method, you simply need to leave the crystals under the light of the sun or the moon for a few hours. For sunlight cleansing, you can simply leave the crystals for 12 hours at a place that gets ample sun. Be aware, however, that some delicate crystals like amethyst shouldn't be exposed to direct sunlight for too long as it can cause discoloration and loss of physical properties. The other method is to leave the crystals under the moonlight for cleansing. The direct sunlight or moonlight will cleanse the crystals and charge them with natural energies.

Holding the Crystals Under Yellow Light

You can cleanse and charge your crystals even by holding them under bright yellow light for longer periods. This will also have a cleansing effect.

Here, a word of caution is important. Under direct sunlight or yellow light, some crystals may start acting as a magnifying glass and start a fire. You must keep this point in mind while cleansing them through these methods.

Cleansing Through Brown Rice

The absorption properties of rice are amazing. It can absorb water and moisture to a great extent. Similarly, it can also absorb energies so you can use rice for cleansing your crystals. Take a jar of rice and bury your crystals under the rice. You must ensure that the crystals aren't visible from any side of the jar. Keep them buried in the jar of rice overnight, and the rice will draw out the negative energy from the crystals. Then, simply leaving the crystals in the sunlight for a few hours will be sufficient to recharge them completely. This method works best for crystals with a delicate nature.

Smudging

You can cleanse your crystals by smudging them. Use smoke from a smothering sage bundle or Palo Santo wood and pass the crystals over it several times to cleanse them. The rising smoke takes away the negative energy of the crystal as it dissipates.

Deep Cleansing Through Burying

Earth has been the birthplace of the crystals like all the mortal beings in the world. It is the mother, and it has the power to cleanse everything. If you feel the need to deep-cleanse your crystals, then you can bury them on the earth for a few days. The vibrational energy of the earth will bring them back to their original form. It will cleanse them of all other influences. Burying the crystals for one or two days will be sufficient.

3. Programming the Crystals

Crystals are natural rocks. They are full of radiant energy that can help you. But to use that energy, it is important to establish a connection with the object from which the energy transfer will be initiated. You will have to program the crystals so that you can achieve your goals. Crystals are not man-made programs. You will need to have a connection of energies with them.

Designate a Place

To establish contact with a new object, you must give it the required attention. The presence of other things emitting energy can interfere with this process. The best place to program your crystals will be a room free of electrical appliances emitting any kind of radiation. Even your mobile phone does that. Program your crystals in a room that is empty and free of distractions so that you can focus.

Clean the Place

Cleanliness is very important in this process. A clean room will be the best place to concentrate. If it is not already clean, then first do so.

State Your Objective and Repeat It Several Times

You will have to make your objective clear. State the thing you are trying to achieve again and again. This serves an important purpose. You will be able to make your intentions clear. Clarity of thought will help you on the way. Hold the crystal in your hands and repeat your intent. Focus on it. You will start feeling the connection with the crystal in a few attempts. If you do not, then cleanse the crystals and repeat the process.

Another way of doing this is to gently rub the crystals in your hands and to repeat your desire. The vibrational energy will help you in establishing the contact with the crystals and in programming them. Keep your intentions clear. Do not set unrealistic goals, and speak them clearly. There is no one else to hear them. The message should go loud and clear to the crystals. Mumbling or hesitating will defeat you here.

What was discussed above is the way to connect the crystals with your psyche. It is an important procedure that must be done with complete honesty. You should feel the connection after some time. If you do not feel this connection with the crystals, it is possible that they are not suited to you, and you will have to replace them.

If you are looking to be healed by the crystals, see them as healers. Feel the healing power of those crystals. Feel the energy radiated by them. The stronger you feel this, better the final results will be.

4. Storing the Crystals

These crystals are going to be of great use to you. Showing the same level of respect when storing them as when you're using them will help in increasing your belief in their powers. Although there is no specific need to store the crystals in any particular type of jar or container, the way you store them will still be important. You can store them in a cloth bag after use or place them in any other container. The important thing is to show respect while doing so. This will not only strengthen your belief, but it will also let you benefit from it. Store the delicate ones with care. Ensure that they do not break or get damaged. Keep them at a designated place after use; this will help you find them again for future use easily even as it feeds strength to your trust in them. Follow this process like a ritual. This ensures the regularity of the procedure, which is important for any type of healing.

Chapter 5: Crystal Healing and Opening Chakras

We have now come to the understanding that different crystals have their specific energy fields. The result of the healing will depend on the type of problem you have and the crystal you have chosen. A thorough understanding of the chakras will give you further insight into this. Many physiological, as well as psychological conditions, can be treated by crystals. The key is to choose the right crystal and place it properly.

Choosing the crystal of the right type and color corresponding to the color of the chakra you are addressing will be important here. You must refer to the table given in Chapter 2 for a better understanding of the concept. The correct placement of the crystal on the chakra will help in removing the blockage of energy and in creating a balance of energy. This is an important part of the healing process. It will bring the most satisfactory results.

There are some crystals which you can wear while there are others that will help you better in meditation. Placing the crystals in the right position will also help you release negative energy, and there are several ways that you can take advantage of the transformative energy of the crystals.

Some of them are as follows:

Wearing Crystals

Some crystals work best when they are placed close to your body. You should be able to feel the vibrations as the crystals rest against your skin. They should remain in contact with the skin. You can wear such crystals as pendants and rings. Keeping them in your pocket would also have a strong impact. If you are impulsive, have anger management issues, or want help in boosting your confidence, wearing such crystals will be of great help.

Holding Crystals While Meditating

Crystals can help you in meditation. Simply holding them in your hands while you meditate will increase your focus, and you will be able to get great results. They have a very soothing effect. You do not need to do anything special. Hold the crystals gently in your hands and start meditating. The energy radiated by the crystals will have a soothing effect on you.

Placing the Crystals on Your Chakras

If there is an energy imbalance in your chakra, then placing specific crystals on their corresponding chakra points will have a superb impact. The crystals will be able to influence the chakras in a better way. They will be able to channel negative energy out and infuse positive energy into your chakras. This will create the required energy balance in the chakras. It doesn't have any negative impact. Your chakras will come together in harmony, and this will have a very positive effect on your health.

In case you are suffering from any disease and are experiencing pain, placing the crystal on the chakra point of that problem will help in easing that pain. It will also help in reducing the impact of the disease on you. For instance, if you are suffering from migraines, placing the crystals on your Third Eye Chakra will help ease them. You can do the same in the case of other ailments, such as stomach disorders, hypertension, or back pain.

Crystals open and activate the chakra points, which can start the self-healing procedure. Our body has a very strong self-healing mechanism. At times, it gets overpowered by sudden and serious illnesses, chronic inflammations, poor lifestyle choices, or improper diet. Once the chakra points open and get activated, they can overpower most of these problems to a great extent.

Depending upon your receptiveness, the nature of the illness, and the kind of power required, you may need to place more than one crystal in a grid form. This will help in radiating the correct level of energy. Different crystals placed in strategic positions will target specific chakras and put them in motion.

It will give a great energy boost to your body. You will feel light, healed, and energetic.

Placing several crystals in a grid form should only be learned in the presence of experts. Wrong selections or placements can create energy imbalance as well. If you are not sure of the number of crystals or of the grid position to be used, restrict yourself to the placing of individual crystals on the chakra points.

Crystal Layout

This is a simple crystal layout for restoring the energy balance in the body. You can do it for yourself or help others with it. Use quartz stone for this process as it works well with all chakras. Choose the color of the quartz crystals according to the color of the chakra you will be placing them on.

1. Prepare the Place

You must lay down on comfortable bedding or cushions and relax. A relaxed mind and body are very important to facilitate a smooth flow of energy. Ensure that the practitioner has lain down properly without facing discomfort.

2. Prepare an Outer Grid

Place the outer grid first. Take four quartz crystals and place one at the head side, one at the feet, and one each at sides of both shoulders.

3. Place the Crystals on the Chakra Points

Now, beginning from the head, place the seven colored crystals on the corresponding chakra points of the practitioner. The selection of color is important here—each crystal's color should correspond to the color of the chakra it's to be placed on, as this ensures better conduction of energy.

4. Point the Crystals Upward

Place all the crystals such that they're pointing upwards. This will ensure the flow of energy from the root chakra to the crown chakra.

5. Visualize the Flow of Energy

The practitioner must visualize the color of every crystal and the corresponding chakra point. This will charge and activate that chakra. Soon the practitioner can feel the surge in his/her energy levels. This will unblock the chakras and also create the energy balance. The practitioner must lie in this position for a few minutes and meditate.

You can practice this energy grid safely on your own. It has a very strong calming effect.

Crystal Grids

Another popular way of healing with crystals is through using a crystal grid. By placing crystals in a powerful geometric pattern that concentrates their vibrations and invoking their energy through affirmations, you direct their influence towards a specific goal, such as curing your back pain or improving your diet.

1. Setting Up the Foundation

Crystal grids manifest the power of sacred geometry. One of the best grids you can use is the Flower of Life, which is shown below. You can print this pattern out or you can look for similar patterns online.

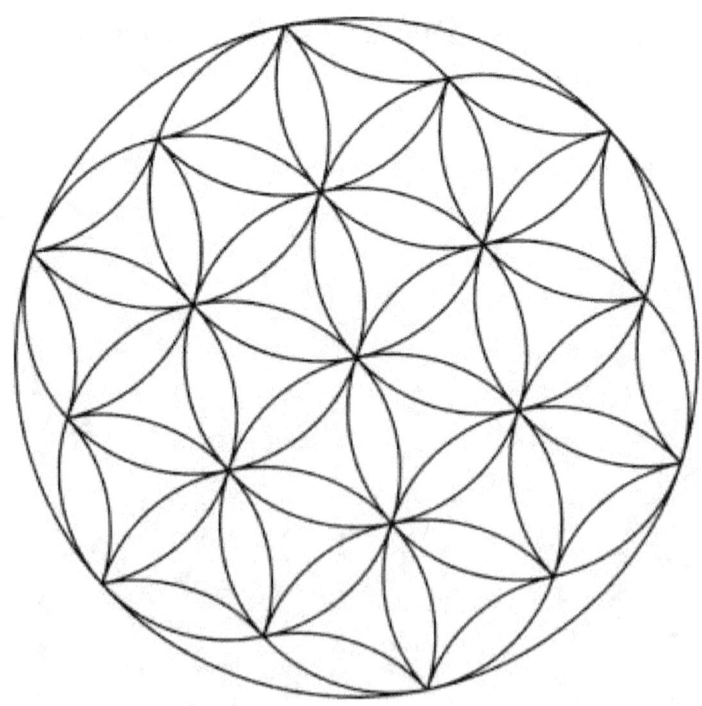

Once you have this pattern printed out and enlarged to fit your needs, choose the proper stones for your purpose. You can use as many or as few stones as you feel necessary but keep a clear, Quartz crystal point to activate your grid.

2. Writing Out Your Affirmation

On a piece of paper, write out your goal and what you want to achieve. Be positive and creative in what you want. For example, to cleanse your aura, remove negative energy, and heal your spirit, you can write, "I am a being of light and hope. Let all negativity drain away. Let my spirit be joyous and filled with healing energy."

3. Cleanse Your Space

Once set up, you want your crystal grid to be undisturbed for 40 days. Therefore, find a place where you can set up your crystal grid. Cleanse that space by smudging it with burning sage.

4. Choosing Your Stones

Select the stones you want to use in your crystal grid. Try not to choose too many, as that will add confusion to your message. You want to focus your intent as much as possible. Select a foundation stone, which should be larger than the rest. Then select 3 different kinds of stones to serve as surrounding stones. You will also need your Quartz crystal to activate your crystal.

To continue our example, our foundation stone will be Aventurine, for cleansing. Our surrounding stones will be Agate to release negativity, Rose Quartz for self-love, and Citrine for healing. We will need two of each surround stone.

In <u>Chapter Six</u>, you will find a list of popular crystals for creating your crystal grid.

5. Laying Out Your Crystal Grid

Place the Flower of Life grid on the space you have chosen. Read out your affirmation and think about how much you want this to happen. Place your folded affirmation in the center of your grid.

Add your surrounding crystals around the center stone, starting from the edge and working inward. You can use multiples of the same stone to create a pleasing effect and to increase their energy. Remember why you choose these stones as you place them.

Sink the foundation stone over your affirmation and meditate on your affirmation.

6. Activate Your Crystal Grid

Activate your crystal grid with your Quartz crystal point by touching each and every crystal, starting from the outside surrounding stones and working your way in. Take a moment to breathe and center yourself. Contemplate the energy of your intention and visualize it being manifested. Imagine your goal completed and the energy of the crystal grid working on your behalf.

Chapter 6:
30 Popular Crystals and Their Healing Properties

Amethyst

This crystal has a very soothing effect. You can use it for meditation as it increases optimism and prevents negativity. It strengthens intuitive powers, and this is one reason it is highly favored by psychics. It also helps in curing emotional blocks. If you are suffering from problems like arthritis and migraine, this is also a must-have for you.

Agate

This crystal helps in the release of negative energy. Whether you are troubled by physical, mental, or spiritual strains, this crystal will help in easing them. If you are troubled by temperamental issues or if some form of addiction is causing problems in your life, this stone can help you a lot as well.

Aquamarine

This crystal helps in overcoming fears. It is best for relieving psychological tensions, stress disorders, panic attacks, and anxiety. People with neurological disorders can receive great help from this crystal.

Aventurine

This is a cleansing crystal. It can clean your body and calm your emotions. You can also add it to your bath water to get relief from anxiety and have a better rest.

Beryl

This crystal helps in treating eye diseases and glandular inflammations. People suffering from colorectal cancer can also get relief from this crystal.

Blue Lace Agate

This crystal has a soothing effect and will help promote clear communication and your receptiveness to higher awakening. It proves confidence and articulation as well as support and resonates well with the throat chakra.

Bloodstone

This crystal has a great impact on improving blood circulation. It helps in cleaning the bloodstream and in keeping you healthy.

Chrysocolla

This crystal offers a great boon to expecting mothers. It helps in easing labor and also cures problems related to the female reproductive system.

Citrine

This crystal helps heal emotional wounds and can be good for recovery after emotional trauma.

Calcite

This crystal can help one get over traumatic experiences of the past. It keeps the chakras in balance and controls rapid heartbeat.

Carnelian

This crystal helps in energizing your body and spirit. If you suffer from lethargy, this is the crystal for you. It also enhances your creativity and sensuality.

Chalcedony

This crystal helps in easing problems caused by mental stress like depression. People suffering from problems like gallstone and blood cancer can also get great help from it.

Chrysoprase

This crystal can ease arthritic pain caused by gout and can also help improve the reproductive health of both the genders.

Citrine

This crystal is the harbinger of luck and success. It boosts your self-confidence and brings fortune. Bearing it in your person will bring luck in business and ward off problems in the vital organs. It keeps the mental condition stable and is especially very helpful for people suspected of doing self-harm.

Diamond

This is one of the most expensive stones in world. Apart from its value in terms of money, it helps in curing diseases of the pineal and pituitary glands. It also reduces toxicity in the body.

Emerald

Yet another precious stone, it helps in treating psychological disorders and makes you more receptive.

Fluorite

This crystal plays a very important role in improving one's powers of concentration and dissolving negative energy. If you are suffering from a lack of focus, then this is the crystal for you. Apart from that, it also helps in curing diseases affecting your bones.

Garnet

This powerful crystal, among other things, helps in restoring hormonal balance in the body.

Hematite

This crystal wards off negative energy. It lowers your stress levels and helps in purifying your blood.

Jade

This crystal infuses ambition. It also helps in curing thyroid problems and diseases affecting the vital organs.

Kunzite

If you are troubled by addictions and are unable to quit them, this crystal can help in strengthening your resolve. It also helps in overcoming schizophrenia.

Malachite

This crystal helps in balancing your left and right brain and keeps them coordinated. It improves your eyesight and also helps in improving your relationships.

Pyrite

This crystal helps in purifying the respiratory tract and also improves digestion. Pyrite also helps with manifesting your intentions and goals.

Quartz

Quartz is the one of the most powerful healing crystals in existence. Made from silica, it encourages overall health and healing. It also helps amplify the strength of other healing crystals and serves to rebalance and recharge your personal energy field.

Red Jasper

If you suffer from digestive tract infections very frequently, then wearing this crystal can be greatly beneficial. It very good for protection and vitalit.

Rose Quartz

Rose quartz is good for love and generosity. This crystal brings Divine love, self-love, and emotional healing. It promotes harmony, trust, and self-care.

Ruby

This crystal is a boon for the Heart Chakra. It also harmonizes your emotional desires and spiritual goals.

Smoky Quartz

This stone is wonderful for shielding and cleansing one of negative and unwanted energy. It helps you let go of outdated beliefs and behaviors.

Turquoise

This crystal helps in healing the Throat Chakra, facilitating communication, and also does a commendable job in hiding the early signs of aging.

Topaz

This crystal increases your appetite and also plays a crucial role in fighting tuberculosis.

Chapter 7:
Maintenance of Crystals

Crystals are delicate in nature. Most crystals are brittle, and lack of care will not only make them dull but also pose a danger of damage. Careless handling of the crystals will not only mean the loss of investment but of time as well.

You must keep in mind some important things to keep your crystals in perfect shape.

Clean Carefully

Washing the crystals under running water and swabbing them with a dry cloth is a good cleaning procedure. But this alone may not suffice at times. Crystals with sharp edges and difficult-to-clean corners can accumulate dust deposits. Cleaning them with soft cleaning agents once in a while is good. However, while cleaning the crystals, you must ensure safe handling.

Packing

You do not need specific packing boxes for many crystals, but keeping the delicate ones with other crystals may cause damage. Keep the delicate ones in glass boxes to avoid such problems.

Place

You will need the crystals on a regular basis; therefore, keeping them at a fixed place is always a good idea. However, they should be kept out of the reach of young children as there is always a danger of accidental choking.

Cleaning Material

Freshwater is good for cleaning crystals. But washing crystals using hot water will always involve risk—some crystals will break when treated with it.

Conclusion

Thanks again for taking the time to download this book! You should now have a good understanding of healing with crystals, and be able to address many common ailments.

If you enjoyed this book, please take the time to leave me a review on Amazon. I appreciate your honest feedback, and it really helps me to continue producing high-quality books.

For further information, here are a couple of books that I found to be extremely useful in developing my understanding of crystal healing.

- *Crystal Enlightenment: The Transforming Properties of Crystals and Healing Stones (Crystal Trilogy, Vol. 1)* by Katrina Raphaell
- *The Magic And Science Of Jewels And Stones...* by Isidore Kozminsky
- *The Healing Power of Gemstones: In Tantra, Ayurveda, and Astrology* by Harish Johari

About the Author

Miriam Petersen is a life-long seeker of knowledge who discovered alternative healing and the path to inner peace in 2013 after struggling with depression and anxiety. As she continued her journey into awakening her higher consciousness, she learned to mute her inner critic and embraced positivity as a life philosophy. She continues to explore different ideas of self-care and healing through meditation, yoga, crystals, light therapy, aromatherapy, and self-hypnosis.